Don't Die By Your Own Hands!

A Busy Person's Guide
to
Overcoming Emotional Eating

Reeshemah Holmes

The information in this book is not intended to serve as medical advice. This book is for educational and informational purposes only.

Requests for permission, speaking engagements and other inquiries should be addressed to:

FIT 4 Success, LLC
4008 Louetta Road, Suite 190
Spring, Texas 77388
Phone: (866) 206-3886

Email: Info@AmericasTopHealthCoach.com

Website: AmericasTopHealthCoach.com

Book Coaches: Jacqueline Escalante Deas and Dawniel Patterson Winningham

Editor: Veronica Allen

This book is written for all the people who are just like me five years ago:

You are suffering from chronic health issues due to subpar personal choices, unhealthy food intake and an overextended lifestyle.

Scariest of all: Going to the doctor month after month because you know you don't feel "right", yet the solutions offered are more testing, medications and possibly surgeries.

This book is for you! Below I am including 2 quotes that caused me to stop dying by my own hands.

ROMANS 14:20 (New Living Translation) states: **Do not forsake the work of God for the sake of food.**

The Dalai Lama stated that what surprised him most about humanity is: ***"Man. Because he sacrifices his health in order to make money. Then he sacrifices money to recuperate his health. And then he is so anxious about the future that he does not enjoy the present; the result being that he does not live in the present or the future; he lives as if he is never going to die, and then dies having never really lived."*** – Dalai Lama

DEDICATION

Thank you to my husband and best friend, Nathan who has supported me while I have journeyed to find my true purpose in life and learn to be good to myself.

Hugs and sweet kisses to the legacy that Nathan and I have created in Nariah and Nathan II. You have taught me to give up the notion of being superwoman or even supermom. This has made our lives more relaxing and much more fun.

ACKNOWLEDGMENTS

Thank you to my mom, Marvis Stewart Bell, for investing time, energy and money into the best educational resources for me. You have always been an excellent role model for healthy living.

Thank you to Oman Jones, for investing time into my understanding of nutrition and the power of all foods. You were a catalyst for sparking my interest in health coaching and I am eternally grateful for you.

Thank you to my fitness trainer, Phillip Fontenot for being one of the most skilled fitness trainers in Houston. I'm still amazed that you can have 10 clients in the gym training with 10 different workouts. You are amazing!

Thank you to Dr. Ian Smith, for creating The Fat Smash Diet. It was my pure joy to finally discover food choices and exercise plans that were flexible and gave me the results I desired at a steady pace.

Thank you to Jimmie Lee for introducing me to Juice Plus. You could be my mother in age, yet we are truly sisters! It's my honor and blessing from God to share the power of foods to the world with you.

Special thanks and love to my clients. I could not have done this without your amazing transformations.

Thank you and much love to my business colleagues, "Natural Weight Loss Coach" Facebook page friends and everyone who has encouraged me along the way. You know who you are!

FOREWORD

My "Wake Up Call" came from Coach Reeshemah

As a coach it is my job to ensure that my clients are not only true to their dream, but they must also be true to themselves as they work towards capturing the dream.

I often encounter clients who want to change, they really do, but in order to change they must face a stark reality about themselves; they must face the reality that they NEED to change.

It was Reeshemah that helped me to face this stark reality about myself. Remember here again, I am a coach. As a coach I am most often on the delivering end of stark realities that other individuals are hiding behind that is keeping them from being successful. Reeshemah helped me uncover a stark reality about myself that was threatening my very life.

As humans we only have so much time in the day and it becomes easy for us to shift other priorities well ahead of taking care of ourselves. We use the kids, the husband, our jobs, and other seemingly valid reasons to avoid the fact that if we don't take care our health then it is all for nothing.

When speaking to Reeshemah about my weight (and the fact that too much of it existed) I presented her with many excuses that were preventing me from taking charge with my health and with my eating. I told her simply that I was too busy making an existence to take time out to do the things that she was suggesting.

That is when she hit me with a bombshell. She told me this: *"Look in the mirror and ask yourself, Are you willing to die by your own hand*? Are you willing to be the one responsible for taking YOU away from your family? Yes you are earning money and making an existence for them now, but what happens when YOU are no longer here because you did not make YOUR HEALTH a priority."

No I didn't instantly change that day. But the words she spoke grew like a seed within me. If I could ignore the thoughts during my waking hours, they served to take over during my slumber. I had nightmares of my overweight corpse being lowered into the ground and my children asking GOD why, for him only to tell them that it was ME that had caused this early death. So I woke up. Not "woke up" in the literal sense meaning from that dream, but instead "woke up" to what was needed for me to get into shape. I have since started a health and fitness plan and it takes priority over EVERYTHING else in my life. Because if I have no life, then I would have no need for those priorities.

I won't say it is easy to start a health and fitness plan. I have years of habits that I must work to overcome to stay on this road. Sometimes I fall off the wagon all together. At those times I must remember the words of Reeshemah. I look in the mirror and I ask myself with all honesty. "Are you willing to die by your own hands?" To which I answer no, and quietly and humbly go somewhere and climb right back onto my wellness plan.

Dawniel Patterson Winningham is a successful corporate and master life coach, award winning speaker, best-selling author and founder of National Day of Sisterhood: (www.nationaldayofsisterhood.com.

You can visit her on the web at www.dawnielwinningham.com for updates on her current health situation.

She is currently eating to live as opposed to living to eat.

CONTENTS

INTRODUCTION

This book was created to serve as a healthy living and weight loss guide to give you control of your own health.

Medical professionals as well as health and fitness professionals can be confident in trusting this lifestyle guide to provide the emotional support needed for health and wellness plans.

The key points in this guide and the accompanying journal will apply to any food plan you may be enjoying at this time. Both resources will serve as a gentle reminder of what is required to improve your health and/or weight loss goals by overcoming emotional eating.

To access your **free 30 Day POWER Lifestyle Journal** visit AmericasTopHealthCoach.com.

With all the articles, recipes and food plans we have access to, it's shocking that our health is failing at an epidemic rate.

This book is for the person who is as tired of going to the doctor as I was; Frustrated at being encouraged for prescriptions and surgeries, yet no one ever cared about identifying the root of the cause to prevent it from returning.

The end result is the same. With this book you have everything you need to change your mindset, change your habits and finish what you start!

CHAPTER 1

WHY ARE YOU DOING THIS?

"You don't have to be great to start, but you must start to be great." – Zig Ziglar

Here you are once again, ready to begin another diet. You are busy as ever; yet your goal is still the same**: end emotional eating and lose weight**. Today, there may be many reasons why you are determined NOT to die by your own hands because of your food choices:

- Your doctor has suggested you lose weight;
- Your clothes fit too tight;
- You are physically tired; and/or
- All of the above plus more!

Relationship Between Your Weight & Your Mind

Emotional eating involves turning to food to suppress or soothe negative emotions, such as stress, anger, fear, boredom, sadness and loneliness. Both major life events and the hassles of daily life can trigger negative emotions that lead to emotional eating and disrupt your healthy living efforts. These triggers may include:

- Health issues
- Career issues
- Financial issues
- Relationship conflicts
- Fatigue

Numerous studies have shown how emotional eating wreaks havoc on any sensible food plan.

Pick any of the emotions or situations above and the fact still remains that emotional eating serves as a form of procrastination. In fact, I often tell my clients that emotional eating is not a solution. If it was, then they should not eat their food; they should pray to it!

With this guide, you are well on your way to investing the energy in yourself to identify what is really eating at you. Meaning, what you ***loose*** in your mind, you will inevitably ***lose*** in your body!

The Power of a Food Journal

Reaching your health goal and maintaining it is a process that requires time to track what progressive and deterring trends you notice in your overall lifestyle habits. Creating healthy habits and maintaining your health is something no one else can do for you. You are going to have to muster up the strength within yourself, stay focused and do what needs to be done to receive the results you desire!

So, what is it going to take to make this lasting change? It will require mastery of **The POWER Lifestyle** program which is outlined step by step in this guide and based on **daily accountability**.

I created **The POWER Lifestyle** 30 day program and it is an acronym for "**People of Wisdom Eating Right**". What makes **The POWER Lifestyle** different from other accountability plans is the fact that your focus will **not** be solely on food, but yourself, your lifestyle and your relationship with God. **The POWER Lifestyle** includes journaling food intake consumption, charting your daily results, moving more and surrounding yourself in healthy relationships during a 30 day time period. No matter how much weight you have to lose, focusing on the next 30 days is an important part of your internal growth. Don't stop reading here! I know it may sound like a lot to start, but trust me, you are worth it!

Before we get to the nuts and bolts of The POWER Lifestyle, there are 3 important points to remember:

1: You know exactly what is required to lose physical weight: Eat fruits and veggies, drink water, exercise, sleep more and stress less. So there you have it! Regardless of the exercise plan you follow and the food plan you decide to select, your personal mental power has to be restored. Remember, you are the only person who puts food in your mouth!

2: You control how you look at feel: Losing weight has to do with sacrifice and discipline. Your "sacrifice" will be a direct correlation to your level of success with your weight loss. You will discover what needs to be sacrificed in your life when you begin to pay attention to your habits. This is one reason why charting and journaling is a must.

It's important to focus on how **you look** and not everyone else. When you see people in magazines or before/after pictures on the internet, this could be you too, if you want it bad enough. What you must stop doing is comparing yourself to other people unless you personally know them, because you have no idea of their daily regimen. Some people take fat burners, risky supplements and others simply workout 3-4 hours a day, 6 days a week. Unless you are willing to give up what they sacrificed to look the way they do, stay engulfed in your own life for now and learn to master **The POWER Lifestyle** for yourself.

3: There are thousands of diets that exist and all of them work for one reason or another.

Nutrition is a major factor in weight loss and healthy living. You may even find that most of these food plans are even comparable with just a few slight differences. The key is to select a food plan (as I like to call it instead of diet), that works for your budget, lifestyle and includes foods that you enjoy eating. As a Health Coach one of my primary responsibilities involves creating food plans to maximize my client's time, money and energy. If you are interested in selecting the best options for your food plans, contact my office directly at AmericasTopHealthCoach.com for a phone consultation. Your success will either arrive early or elude you based on how much you decide to follow the food plan you select.

To prove this point, one day while standing in the store checkout line, I noticed that three out of ten magazine covers highlighted articles on getting rid of belly fat. I became curious to the solution they offered. After spending 5 minutes reading the articles, they all said basically the same thing:

- Eliminate sugars
- Reduce stress
- Exercise
- Eat lean proteins
- Eat fruits and veggies

That's it! Each article added their own spin to "the how" of achieving these 5 steps and voila! Another cover story is purchased AND another food plan is started, although perhaps never finished.

As we end this chapter I want you to be crystal clear on two facts:

- **Time is of the essence**! Whether you stay engaged in **The POWER Lifestyle** or not, the 30 day mark will come! How you feel about yourself and your results will be indicative of what you decide to do on a daily and maybe even hourly basis.
- **This is a lifestyle management book, not just another diet or food plan.** This book has been created to remove all the fluff, marketing and false promises that have left you feeling deflated, remorseful and maybe even caused you to gain weight in the past.

The POWER Lifestyle 30 day program is simple and it works!

CHAPTER 2

HOW BUSY ARE YOU?

A person who wants something will find a way. A person who does not will find an excuse. - Unknown

I know exactly how you feel. You believe you don't have enough time, money or both to provide excellent care for your health. The truth is everyone has the same 24 hours. It is simply a matter of what activities are placed into that time frame on a daily basis.

For this reason, start today to put yourself on your own calendar so that you will consciously learn to do something different to show that you are actively doing your part to live longer. Otherwise, you will forget! You will forget to eat, spend time with God in prayer, meditation, journaling and charting your daily results.

Make Time to Exercise

I have a question for you: Do you exercise?

If not, why not? Exercise has several benefits:

- It helps you lose weight
- Clears your mind
- Curbs food cravings
- Reduces cholesterol
- Keeps your bones strong
- Many more benefits depending on the exercise and the intensity level

When it comes to exercise, some days you simply just do not feel like doing it. After a long day of taking care of everyone else, you are mentally exhausted and simply yearn for peace, quiet and rest. I understand! The irony of being more active in the kitchen and the gym, will show that as you invest time to eating healthy and exercising, you will experience inner satisfaction and peace- yet everything else about your life still remains the same.

Create a Vision for the New You

Now, spend time looking around you. If you have at least one coworker or person in your industry who manages to be healthy, this means you can do it too. If you don't have a physical visual of a person living your desired lifestyle, Google or search the internet to find images of someone who is fit! My point is to show you that **whatever you desire is possible**. Simply make sure that your model is someone with a comparable lifestyle and budget so that you stay encouraged.

Sometimes when you start over with your weight loss goal, especially after you succeed in so many other areas of your life, it seems daunting. This time will be different because you are taking different actions!

NOTE TO SELF: Create Your Affirmation

Write a note to yourself that you will read every morning when you wake up and every night before you go to bed. In the note you will write in detail what you plan to accomplish at the end of the 30 days. Make several copies of this note. Place a copy under your pillow, in your wallet, at your desk, on your refrigerator and anywhere else that you see on a regular basis.

For example, you may write something like this:

My body is renewed and healed as a result of good nutrition. I enjoy drinking water because I understand that it hydrates me and gives me the energy I need to live a powerful life.

I look forward to my 30 minute walks because this is my time of reflection and meditation with God.

The relationships in my life are wholesome. I am growing with people who are good for me and I am also good for them.

My positive self talk keeps me going. I will finish this once and for all and overcome emotional eating by making conscious choices.

Finish What You Start

It is a fact that you are an overachiever and you have accomplished many monumental tasks in your life. Now it is time to overcome emotional eating. Before things can be accomplished they must first be seen. That is one of the foundational truths of goal setting. Your goal of overcoming emotional eating must be reviewed on an ongoing basis to remind you exactly why you are spending this time, effort and maybe occasional frustration to reach the goals that you have set for yourself. If you are indeed determined to finish what you start, here are 3 points to implement: visualization, setting realistic goals and managing your goals.

Your 30 Day Commitment

The POWER Lifestyle makes you aware of your life again and you now have the ability to consciously take full control of your actions. Here is the ultimate truth: 30 days can sometimes feel like 30 months when you are creating new habits. You may find that focusing on just one day at a time is the way to go for you. In this case, a short term goal for you will be one hour and a long term goal will be one day.

Every day you will complete your **POWER Lifestyle** activities: tracking and analyzing the time you spend x 30 days will equal your goal. You still have the same 30 day goal, yet you broke it down into a time system that is easier for your mind to digest. This process of focusing on one hour and one day at a time to complete 30 day goal(s) is exactly how I was able to finally complete a lifestyle overhaul that I desperately craved.

Contract with Yourself

Completing **The POWER Lifestyle** program is an agreement solely with yourself and the rewards are increased awareness , better health, hydrated body, more energy, restful sleep and reciprocal relationships, just to name a few.

Your compliance with **The POWER Lifestyle** is also a reflection of your personal character and accountability to yourself. Character has to do with who you are when no one is watching. Yes, you are extremely busy, many people rely on you, and for one reason or another you have not given yourself the attention that is needed to live your best life possible. All of this is changing right now. To make a definitive decision and move forward, I want you to determine if you are giving yourself reasons to excel or excuses to stall.

REASONS VS EXCUSES

There is a difference between a reason and an excuse. A reason is a justifiable cause. An example of a reason is you are late going to the gym or you don't show up at the gym because your flight is delayed. That's a valid reason. However, if you are traveling, tired when you landed and decided to go to bed early, that's an excuse. An excuse is something you tell yourself why you are not doing what you know you should be doing.

The next 30 days you will push yourself in your mind beyond what you may believe you are able to achieve. You are an overachiever for the next 30 days! You are indeed busy and it's time to show up and be busy for yourself. **No more excuses are allowed**.

Goal Snatchers

What lifestyle situations ultimately cause you to emotional eat? Perhaps:

- You are busy
- You work 80 hours a week
- You are tired
- You are sleepy
- You are traveling
- You don't know what to eat
- You are lonely, sad or happy
- You are a social eater/drinker

- You can't say no
- You are depressed/ stressed

THESE ARE ALL EXCUSES!

It is now time to focus on yourself! You have done something great by taking the first step to invest in this guide. Now become even greater by adjusting your mindset and habits to actively finish **The POWER Lifestyle** 30 day program.

Remember, stay consciously in charge of the direction that your thoughts take you. For the next 30 days commit to following **The POWER Lifestyle** 100% and you will be amazed at what happens when you finish what you start.

This 30 day lifestyle program is the solo game of you creating and living your best life. Every entry in the companion journal, shows a page in your mosaic life. To achieve the goals you set, you must fully participate and you must show up and give what is required to receive what you desire in every area of your life.

When you become determined to do what you can to live as long as possible, you will experience a better quality of life.

Are you willing to have someone wiping your butt in a few decades because you could not control the foods you put in your mouth?! This is what you have to ask yourself and think about.

Today you are in control of every choice you make to serve you well, or work total opposite against you.

At the end of each chapter answer the following questions in your journal:

- *What have I learned about my habits in this chapter?*
- *What other areas of my life are my habits overflowing into?*
- *Who else do my habits (good or bad) directly affect?*

CHAPTER 3

MIND OVER MATTER:

The power of prayer AND meditation

"Prayer is when you talk to God. Meditation is when you listen to God". - The People's Almanac

This is a foundational chapter for **The Power Lifestyle**. Reread this chapter as needed to create a strong foundation to end emotional eating.

Ten Steps of The Power Lifestyle

To be successful in **The POWER Lifestyle**, there are ten steps for you to implement and master:

1: Your POWER lifestyle mindset

No matter what you say, no one knows what you are thinking. It is up to you to control your thoughts, because your thoughts determine your actions and your actions determine the result you will receive from this program and life. Your current mindset is based on beliefs and traditions which may have been passed down for generations! You have simply lived the way that you were taught. You may have new healthy habits to learn simply because no one introduced them in a way that would work for you.

Child/Adult Mentality

Every person has a child and an adult mentality.

The focus that you place on recognizing whether you currently have a child or adult mentality will be a foundational step for success in every area of your life including: Your career, relationships, finances, self value and healthy living goals.

The child mentality seeks instant gratification and is selfish. It is also irresponsible and has no qualms about not reaching goals because this mentality believes in living in the moment.

The adult mentality is responsible, reliable and understands the value of patience. This mindset is also determined to finish a task that is started.

Both of these mindsets vie for control of your focus. People often wonder which one has control. The answer is, the one you cater to the most. The one you focus on and allow to have their way.

Tony Robbins says *"You can never achieve anything significant in life without a behavior change* ***and*** *a mental shift".*

In addition to this, I lean towards the coaching of Dawniel Patterson Winningham:

"If changing was that simple and you could do it by yourself, you would have done it a long time ago."

2: Your Habits

There may be habits you have that were passed down from your great -great grandparents simply by word of mouth and no one has ever changed it. One example I can give you is when people say "Everyone in my family is overweight". Actually, it may be that everyone in your family eats unhealthy food on a regular basis and doesn't place a high priority on being physically active.

Now you will begin to clearly see in black and white exactly what you repeatedly do. For some people it may not always be eating unhealthy; they may not eat at all by skipping meals. Other people eat healthy, yet lack in being physically active.

Regardless of what needs to be tweaked with your 30 Day POWER Journal, your lifestyle choices will now be right in front of you to be addressed and positively altered.

3: Your Emotions

The #1 cause of obesity is emotional eating. Weight gain doesn't always stem from what you are eating, but what is eating at you.

As mentioned earlier, emotional eating is a coping mechanism for dealing with negative emotions. Instead of facing the causes of stress, anger, sadness or anxiety directly, you soothe or comfort yourself with food. But after the initial pleasure from eating dissipates, the emotions that triggered the craving still remain. Nothing has been done to rectify or remedy the emotional state, and you often feel worse than before. Emotional eating stems from an emotional hunger. In essence, you use food to fill a void that is reserved for God.

Emotional eating can also be difficult to treat. The Mayo Clinic suggests trying self care methods before seeking professional help. A large part of self healing involves changing how you see, speak and feel about yourself. If you look in the mirror, call yourself fat and can't stand how you look, it becomes true because you said it. You will have to make up your mind to see the best in yourself, the same way I bet you see the best in others.

4: Your Perceptions

Perhaps you were never taught the importance of health growing up. Maybe you were an athlete, yet never learned the role nutrition played in performance. In both instances, your perception involved the things that you believed to be true, whether it is based on facts or not. It also has to do with your experiences and belief system. This goes back to your childhood teachings, your experiences and your emotional stability.

As the overachiever, it is sometimes comforting to see others succeed or maybe to feel "needed" for one reason or another. Over time, your habits caused you to push your own personal needs, wants and desires further and further down the line for your attention. This will now change.

5: Your Strategies

When aiming to finish any project, time and energy is invested into how to reach the end result. Many times adding in how to finish in the shortest amount of time and spending the least amount of money. This is directly tied to strategies and tactics.

Strategies are the game plan of success.

For example your POWER Lifestyle strategies would involve asking yourself the following questions:

- *What food plan am I going to follow?*
- *How am I going to eat 5 fruits and 5 veggies daily?*
- *How am I going to get in daily exercise?*

The POWER Lifestyle tactics are the actions that will be required to take the steps such as:

- waking up earlier to exercise and prepare meals
- exercising during lunch
- exercising during kid appointments

- eating before you go on appointments or errands and
- prepping and preparing food in advance

Now, we must tackle the biggest why of all:

<u>Why do you do the things that you do?</u>

Start asking yourself this question daily and in every realm of your life.

Also ask yourself:

- Why am I going out of my way to eat 5 fruits and 5 veggies daily? (NOTE: May need to be adjusted for medical reasons)
- Why is it important for me to complete this 30 Day POWER Lifestyle program?
- Why am I making myself wake up early to pray, meditate and spend time with God?

6: Your SYSTEMS

SYSTEM means **Save Yourself Some Time, Energy and Money.** Yes, you may have invested in this guide, but I am pushing you to finish **The**

POWER Lifestyle program as created because it works and it gives you freedom to live your life!

Freedom also includes adjusting your food or exercise plan as needed to fit your lifestyle - yet staying focused on your end result. By sticking to **The POWER Lifestyle**, you may find yourself saving a significant amount of money on food. You can use these funds for non food rewards such as massages, kitchen gadgets, exercise gear, support groups, additional coaching, etc.

You are now beginning the habit of actively living your best life and ending the cycle of living on autopilot!

7: YOUR HONESTY

It is time to face the truth: You are the only person who can make you healthy. You are also solely responsible for keeping yourself sick from preventable diseases. Every time you bring something to your mouth, whether it is coffee, cigarettes, sugars, veggies, fruits, water, candies, smoothies, salads, chips, breads, diet drinks and everything in between, I want you to decide today to make conscious decisions.

Stop and ask yourself:

"Is this going to help me reach my goals?" before putting it in your body. From that point, make a conscious choice to improve your health and/or reach your goals.

Stop. Pause. Think.

Is this something that will serve you well and be a glowing example of what God wants for you?

No, I am not saying don't ever eat cheese steaks, popcorn, ribs, red velvet cake, etc. I am suggesting you make conscious decisions. Eat your food slow, enjoy it and make sure you burn it off in exercise.

Determine in your mind once and for all, that you deserve the best of everything - especially food.

For example, restaurant and fast foods taste great but they are normally shockingly high in sodium, sugar, fat and calories. Therefore, when eating outside your home or at events, scan the food to determine if you see something that you really want **and** that is good for you. If possible, search for fruits, veggies and even consider asking for a special request! Don't waste your energy on foods that contain empty calories.

Instead, eat the absolute best choices, eat half of your normal portion and eat it slowly.

8: Learn how to give 100% daily

Do not start with trying to give 100% for 30 days. Focus on giving 100% for 3 days only. Verbally affirm **"I am going to give 100% to myself, to God and my commitment to my life**." When those 3 days are over, commit for another 3 days. Repeat this new habit 10 times and that's an entire month. This will motivate you because you can do anything for 3 days!

During this process, you will be honest about your lifestyle choices and go back to review your activities in your 30 Day POWER Lifestyle Journal for daily accountability and also track your daily data to let you know how you are doing.

With **The POWER Lifestyle**, it is important to follow every principle and do your best every day. This lifestyle program will build up your mind, body and spirit to make you a fully energetic person serving yourself and benefitting the world in a wonderful way within a short period of time.

In The POWER Lifestyle program, you will inevitably find a principle that requires extra mental and sometimes physical energy to complete. Remind yourself this learning curve will last as long as it takes you to reach your goal and then you advance to the maintenance phase.

For some people this may be exercise. Thinking about exercise may not motivate you at all, but it must be done. Therefore it helps to rename the exercise and call it something different. Perhaps call it "activity for_____". That blank could be goal weight party, photo shoot, get off high blood pressure medication, etc. You will need to go back to **your why** to fill in this blank.

9: Your Praying

This is the one area that will keep you calm and help to end emotional eating. Yet it's the one area most people forget. Do it!!!!

Find a mantra, scripture and/or quote that touches you in regards to staying focused. Always pray BEFORE you eat also!

Having conversations with God doesn't have to always be an on your knees, eyes closed, hands in the air experience either.

Pray to God when you are in the midst of the foods, places and people that are strongholds in your life. Simply focus in your mind and ask God to help you be good **to** yourself so that you may be good **for** others.

Talk to God as you pass by places and things that are tempting for you. Before you know it, you will feel mentally stronger by placing your challenges in the hands of God. Eventually you will crave the time you set aside to pray and meditate.

As you learn to make conscious choices to overcome your cravings and temptations, you won't feel so physically weak and exhausted either. Instead you will feel strong and powerful because you are building up the stamina in your mind and making yourself mentally and physically stronger.

Peter I 3:3-4 states: *"Your beauty should not come from outward adornment, such as braided hair and the wearing of gold jewelry and fine clothes. Instead, it should be that of your inner self, the unfading beauty of a gentle and quiet spirit, which is of great worth in God's sight."*

Stay engaged! Show up! Perhaps for the first time in a very long time, this is going to be a mosaic time in your life.

10: Your Affirmations

It is said that "You have to see it before you will believe it." Actually, you must believe it before you see it. This is where visualization and written affirmations play a major role in your success.

Written affirmations will assist you in losing weight faster, while eliminating emotional eating, food cravings, resistance to exercise and other mental blocks.

Affirmations work because they are not descriptions of your current situation; they are goals you have already achieved. In other words, they are goals you intend to make come true for you - and it is the power of your intention that fuels the affirmation.

In order to work, affirmation should be:

1. Short, specific and action oriented
2. Written in the positive and present tense
3. Credible, yet still stretch your belief
4. Able to create a feeling inside of you of already reaching your goal weight
5. Repeated at least 10 times daily

6. Activated in your mind as if it's happening now.

Visualization works with pictures and vision boards. Find a favorite picture of yourself so you can remember that you have done this before. If you have not, take a picture of yourself today as a starting point. Find a few bible verses to be inspired by God and you are on your way.

2 Timothy 1:7 is an excellent example to read: "God did not give you a spirit of fear; but of love, **POWER** and self discipline."

Locate a scripture that takes your mind to the highest point to stay close to God - and keep it there. If you are at a point where you feel you are about to break, take the pressure off yourself and pray at that very moment. **God will give you strength that surpasses all understanding.**

CHAPTER 4

CHANGE JUST ONE THING...

"There is nothing wrong with change, if it is in the right direction". - Winston Churchill

Learn to take care of yourself before you take care of anyone else. Period. Until you learn to do this, it will hinder your relationships in one way or another. Even on an airplane, they instruct you to put your mask on first before you assist someone in putting on their mask.

The majority of emotional eaters lead fairly simple lives: They don't drink, smoke, go out often and may not spend money on much, except for food. This is where the food trap comes in, because they start to tell themselves they "deserve" to have enjoyable food.

Exercise is one thing that can be changed.

Remember, what you eat, you must burn off. Therefore, engage in as much physical movement as you can early in the morning because you have no idea what may transpire during the day. If you pack your meals, exercise, pray and meditate in the morning, you have taken care of yourself first.

Your daily tracking in your 30 Day Power Lifestyle Journal will be the constant visual to keep you accountable of your new lifestyle and a check and balance system of what you think and what you actually do.

Acknowledge the areas where you are struggling and seek additional support immediately. This is very important for your progression. Many times it's not that you do not know what to do, you simply have not been shown how to do it in a way that benefits you. That's it!

Journal and Track Your Days

Thoughts disentangle themselves in words and this is the data **your POWER lifestyle** journal provides. Journaling provides healing and therapeutic solutions by transferring the energy from the mind to the paper. You will be able to track different areas of your life and journal your thoughts on a daily basis. Remember that both tracking and journaling are very important for your progression.

Tracking is something you do in other areas of your life. If you sat down with your boss and had no track record of work you completed, would your boss give you a raise or consider you for a promotion?

What if God did that for our lives? What if God said " *I had so much work for you to accomplish on earth, but you couldn't let go of your own selfish desires long enough to receive the blessings and awards."*

I had so much work that I needed for you to complete for me, but you couldn't get out of your own space and stop stuffing your mouth and your body to have the energy to maximize your life. "Would this finally wake you up?

Get a Buddy

To maximize your results even further will involve having an accountability partner or buddy. Select an accountability partner that you send your daily log to every day. One caveat: No exceptions and no lies! This is very important.

With the daily activities in your accompanying journal, by the end of each day, you can see how you completed the tasks that are important to you and served you well.

Within the **POWER Lifestyle** 30 day period, you will learn to appreciate the powerful and divine person that God created you to be. The same way you have your own fingerprint, you also have your own body, life, lifestyle, income, etc. Now is the time to pay attention to everything that is happening to make up YOU!

REFRAIN vs. REPETITION

A big part of **The POWER Lifestyle** is the freedom to eat whatever you like. You just may not be able to eat it every single day, or in the same portion size. So you have to learn how to refrain from unhealthy products (Some things we call food should really be called a product) **and** restrain yourself from your own selfish desires and habits to ultimately reach the goals you have set for yourself.

For example, if you have a desire for carrots,

apricots, bananas, etc. this serves you well! No need to refrain here.

REFRAIN is defined in Webster's dictionary as *"To keep oneself from doing, feeling or indulging in something and especially from following a passing impulse.* The example the dictionary gives is to refrain from having dessert!

Social/emotional eating, on the other hand, has proven to be a habit that requires adequate attention. At your job, in meetings and/or social settings, they may serve all types of pastries and junk food. Before you indulge in this, go to the bathroom or just sit still if you have to and pray to God to give you strength. This takes you out of your own power and builds up your spirit so that you will have the mental and spiritual strength to go back and watch others eat this junk food because you know it does not serve you well.

Psalm 138:3 states:," *When I pray you answer me, you lift me up and give me strength." (New Living Translation)*

Ask yourself on a daily basis:

How am I doing in refraining myself from foods, habits and people that do not serve me well?

REPETITON is defined in Webster's dictionary as "*Doing something over and over again; a motion or exercise that is repeated and usually counted; such as push- ups.*

Refraining and repetition are strongly connected to **rote memorization**: memorization by repetition. It is the process of making decisions without thinking about what we learned early in life. Take notice of what you eat but also where you are, who you are with and intentionally pay attention to the patterns you notice in your life.

As you learn to refrain more, you may find that as the month continues, your stomach may shrink. You will still eat 5-10 fruits and veggies daily but your serving size may become smaller. You will love when this happens!

Questions to ask yourself are:

- What should I refrain from more?
- What can I do to maximize my tracking and journaling?

CHAPTER 5

WHAT ARE YOU EATING?

"Until you value yourself, you will not value your time. Until you value your time, you will not do anything with it."

M Scott Peck

JUNK FOOD: Yes, this word is indeed in Merriam Webster's dictionary with two definitions.

#1: *"Food that is high in calories but low in nutritional content."*

#2:*"Something that is appealing or enjoyable but of little of no real value."*

Did this strike a chord with you?

Have you ever told yourself "I want some junk food?" or you find yourself buying food from a vending machine?

Actually is it even food?

Would it be better just to skip a meal?

I promise you probably will be ok if you skip a meal! You might get a headache. This is not a headache because you are hungry but perhapse due to an imbalance of sugar, salt, caffeine or maybe even toxins that your body is craving.

Can you believe the definitions of FAST FOOD are in the dictionary too? The definitions are:

1: *Specializing in food that can be prepared and served quickly.*

2: Designed for ready availability use or consumption with little consideration given to quality or significance. The 2nd definition was just created in 1951!

Knowing that your body is the temple of God and God resides in you, you are assured that your strength and power comes from God. Would you now choose to feed your body and mind with food that has been created with little consideration for quality?

So again, is it better to eat fast food or skip a meal? This is the time to feed yourself the Word of God!

SUPER FOODS: According to www.helpguide.org, these foods are defined as *"Rich in vitamins and nutrients. Minimally processed foods that provide your body with the maximum amount of nutrition. "*

What would you rather do? Eat super foods or go hungry? Eat super foods!

Super foods are important because they are nutrient dense with vitamins and minerals. Your body was created to keep you alive! The way you can see the real "you" is to analyze your body and listen to your body. Food is fuel for your mind, body and energy. The rest of your body that we see is simply an outward reflection of your habits and choices. That's it.

Your body is so intelligent and magnificent that scientists are still unsure about the full potential of it. If your body is properly fed through nutrition and food, the damaged area can regenerate itself. If your body is not properly fed, it can still function to keep you alive. The only difference is you will feel dehydrated, fatigued and experience something always feeling "off" in your body.

Remember, it is not normal to be tired and have low energy!

You can tell super foods by the color! They look alive: red, orange, pink, yellow, purple, green, and more!

Non superfoods (junk food) are two main colors: brown or white. They have been processed, refined and created by man for two purposes:

1: To sell or make money

2: Get you addicted to junk food

They can normally be found in your pantry and last for months. Non superfoods also have nutritional labels and may cause preventable diseases.

Also, superfoods normally make people feel energetic, while non superfoods are known to make people feel tired and moody.

CHAPTER 6

BIRDS OF A FEATHER, FLOCK TOGETHER

Surround yourself only with people who are going to take you higher. Oprah Winfrey

The above quote is truly worth pondering. Pay attention to the things people say to you when you decide to make yourself better by eating healthy and following **The POWER Lifestyle**.

When people start asking why you are on a diet or trying to lose weight, pay attention. They are telling you something about your relationship with them when they ask questions such as:

- *Are you on a diet?*
- *Are you trying to become a vegetarian?*
- *You already look great. Why are you doing this?*

I'm not suggesting you drop your friends. Keep those friends but also meet new people who enjoy the lifestyle you are moving towards.

You will find that the positive people will take up more time and the toxic people will have less to give and give you less time. Eventually, the toxic friends go away. When you spend time seeking out positive people, you will also become more positive.

Now you have it! **The POWER Lifestyle** program is a system of paying attention to your mindset and your habits. As a result of doing this, you will end emotional eating, maximize your days and grow stronger in your relationship with God, yourself and other people.

Carpe Diem!

ABOUT THE AUTHOR

Reeshemah Holmes is an Author and a highly sought after Speaker based in Houston, Texas.

Reeshemah was certified as a Health Coach from the Dr. Sears Wellness Institute. She has obtained health certifications for Families and Children, Expecting and Nursing Moms, Adults and Seniors. She is one of the top Health Coaches in America.

In addition, Reeshemah is a Certified Professional Coach (CPC) and Certified Advanced Law of Attraction Expert.

Reeshemah became a Health Coach after her own body revolted against her at an accelerated pace.

Diagnosed with high blood pressure, high cholesterol, pre-diabetes, fibroids, migraines, peri-menopause and anxiety attacks - all at the same time - she discovered the healing and equally harmful power of foods. The physical breakdown of Reeshemah's body forced her to alter her habits and mindset. For the first time, she began giving herself the same level of quality attention that she had been giving to others.

Starting a holistic approach to self healing, without the intervention of medicine or surgery spurred her to create **The POWER Lifestyle Program**: A Common Sense Approach to Managing Your Life & Your Health.

POWER is an acronym for "People of wisdom eating right".

Reeshemah has dedicated her life to helping others listen to their bodies, live on purpose and experience authentic abundance.

In her free time, Coach Reeshemah does her best to keep up with her wonderful husband of 17 years, two energetic and busy teenagers and her beloved cane corso dog - who has no clue that he is not a human.

Join Reeshemah and receive your **free 30 Day POWER Journal** at:

Website: AmericasTopHealthCoach.com

Facebook:
Facebook.com/CoachReeshemahHolmes
(The Natural Weight Loss Coach)

Twitter: @CoachReeshemah

NOTES:

NOTES:

NOTES:

Made in the USA
Monee, IL
04 November 2026

67375827R00039